30-DAY MINDFUL EATING CHALLENGE

Transforming Your Relationship with Food

Victoria Charles

Table of Contents

INTRODUCTION

The book "30-DAY MINDFUL EATING CHALLENGE: Transforming Your Relationship with Food" offers a compelling and holistic approach to reshaping the way we interact with food. In a world marked by busy schedules, fad diets, and constant distractions, the concept of mindful eating emerges as a beacon of sanity and balance.

In this fast-paced modern age, where meals are often consumed hastily on the go, the fundamental connection between nourishment and well-being has been compromised. The "30-DAY MINDFUL EATING CHALLENGE" aims to rekindle this connection by inviting readers to embark on a transformative journey that extends beyond mere dietary choices.

The book's premise lies in the practice of mindfulness – the art of being fully present and attuned to the current moment. By applying mindfulness to the act of eating, individuals can not only savor the flavors and textures of their meals but also cultivate a deeper understanding of their body's needs and responses. This shift in focus from mindless consumption to conscious indulgence paves the way for a more balanced and harmonious relationship with food.

Throughout the 30-day journey, readers are gently guided through a series of thought-provoking exercises, meditations, and reflections. These exercises are designed not only to enhance the sensory experience of eating but also to illuminate the emotional triggers, habits, and patterns that often underlie our dietary choices. By addressing these deeper aspects, the book fosters a holistic transformation – one that touches not only the way we eat but also the way we perceive and relate to food.

Whether the reader seeks weight management, improved digestion, or a general sense of well-being, the "30-DAY MINDFUL EATING CHALLENGE" offers a versatile roadmap. Backed by scientific insights into the mind-body connection, this book is more than a challenge; it's an opportunity to cultivate mindfulness, nurture a healthier relationship with food, and ultimately, embark on a journey of self-discovery and positive change.

CHAPTER ONE

The Foundations of Mindful Eating: Nurturing a Holistic Connection with Food

In a world characterized by the hustle and bustle of modern life, the simple act of eating has become a rushed and mindless routine for many. Amidst the whirlwind of responsibilities and distractions, the concept of mindful eating has emerged as a powerful antidote – a practice that invites individuals to reclaim a profound and conscious relationship with the food they consume. By intertwining ancient wisdom with contemporary understanding, mindful eating transcends the realm of diets and quick fixes, offering a holistic approach to transforming our connection with food. This exploration delves into the essence of mindful eating, tracing its origins, delving into its philosophical underpinnings, and illuminating how it has the potential to revolutionize the way we nourish ourselves.

Understanding Mindful Eating

Mindful eating is the art of bringing full awareness to the act of eating. It involves being fully present in the moment, engaging all the senses, and savoring each bite with intention and attention. This practice shifts the focus from the sheer consumption of food to the rich experience of nourishment, fostering a deep appreciation for the flavors, textures, and aromas of the food we eat. Unlike traditional dieting, which often revolves around restriction and external rules, mindful eating encourages individuals to listen to their bodies and cultivate a compassionate understanding of their nutritional needs.

Benefits of Mindful Eating

The benefits of mindful eating extend far beyond the realm of physical health. While weight management and improved digestion are frequently cited advantages, the practice's impact goes deeper, touching emotional, psychological, and even spiritual dimensions. Research indicates that mindful eating can lead to reduced binge eating and emotional eating tendencies, as individuals learn to differentiate between physical hunger and emotional cravings. By fostering a heightened awareness of the body's signals, mindful eating also promotes healthier portion control and a more attuned response to hunger and satiety cues.

Furthermore, mindful eating serves as a gateway to a more harmonious relationship with one's body image and self-esteem. As individuals embrace the philosophy of non-judgmental awareness, they can release the negative self-talk often associated with food choices, ultimately cultivating a sense of self-acceptance and self-compassion. This shift in perspective contributes to reduced stress levels, improved mental well-being, and an overall sense of empowerment and agency over one's choices.

Origins of Mindful Eating

While the concept of mindfulness has its roots in ancient Eastern traditions, the incorporation of mindfulness into eating practices gained prominence in the West during the 20th century. The Vietnamese Buddhist monk Thich Nhat Hanh is often credited with introducing mindful eating to the modern world. His teachings emphasize the interconnectedness of all beings and advocate for a conscious awareness of the sources of our sustenance.

Drawing from mindfulness meditation, Hanh introduced the "Five Contemplations" – a set of reflections to be recited before and after meals. These contemplations encourage gratitude for the food, an awareness of the effort invested in its production, and an acknowledgment of the interconnected web of life that brings sustenance to our tables.

Philosophy Behind Mindful Eating

At the heart of mindful eating lies a profound philosophy that transcends the boundaries of food and extends to life itself. Mindful eating invites us to slow down, reconnect with the present moment, and acknowledge the intricate interdependence of all living beings. This philosophy aligns with Buddhist principles of mindfulness, compassion, and non-violence, as well as with the broader movement towards conscious living.

Transforming Your Relationship with Food

The transformation that mindful eating offers is not a mere shift in dietary habits but a profound change in the way we relate to food, our bodies, and the world around us. By embracing the principles of mindful eating, individuals can experience a renewed sense of agency and empowerment over their choices. The practice encourages us to let go of the external pressures of diet culture and instead turn inward, listening to our bodies' innate wisdom.

Mindful eating also helps break the cycle of guilt and shame often associated with food choices. By practicing non-judgmental awareness, individuals can free themselves from the emotional burdens that have long plagued their interactions with food. This, in turn, fosters a healthier and more balanced approach to eating, one that is rooted in self-care and self-compassion.

In essence, mindful eating invites us to embark on a journey of self-discovery. It urges us to explore the intricate tapestry of our senses, our emotions, and our connections to the world. As we develop this heightened awareness, we become attuned to the subtle nuances of our bodies and the cues they provide. This shift in consciousness paves the way for a more intuitive and harmonious relationship with food – one that is centered on nourishment, gratitude, and a profound sense of presence.

Conclusion

In a world that often encourages mindless consumption and quick fixes, the practice of mindful eating stands as a transformative gateway to a more conscious and compassionate way of nourishing ourselves. Rooted in ancient wisdom and infused with modern insights, mindful eating offers a holistic approach to food that transcends diets and restrictions. By understanding its foundations, embracing its philosophy, and experiencing its benefits, individuals can embark on a journey of profound transformation – one that extends far beyond the plate and touches the core of their being.

CHAPTER TWO

The Science Behind Mindful Eating: Nurturing Well-Being Through Awareness

In the realm of dietary trends and weight management strategies, mindful eating emerges not as a fleeting fad but as a scientifically grounded practice with profound implications for our overall well-being. At its core, mindful eating transcends the boundaries of a simple eating regimen; it represents a transformative approach that hinges on the synergy between our mind and body. Grounded in rigorous scientific research, this practice embodies the harmonious integration of ancient mindfulness principles and modern understanding of human physiology and psychology. This exploration delves into the scientific underpinnings of mindful eating, uncovering how it taps into the mind-body connection, and elucidating the wide-ranging benefits that unfold when mindfulness meets our dining table.

Scientific Backing for Mindful Eating

The effectiveness of mindful eating is not merely anecdotal; it's substantiated by a growing body of scientific research. Numerous studies have delved into the impact of mindfulness on eating behaviors, revealing remarkable correlations between mindful eating and healthier food choices, improved digestion, and emotional well-being.

One study, published in the "Journal of Obesity," investigated the impact of mindfulness-based eating awareness training on binge eating behaviors. The results showcased significant reductions in binge eating episodes, highlighting the practice's potential in addressing impulsive and emotional eating patterns.

Moreover, research conducted at Indiana State University explored the relationship between mindfulness and portion control. The study found that participants who engaged in mindful eating consumed smaller portions compared to those who ate mindlessly. This suggests that mindfulness encourages individuals to tune into their body's signals of hunger and satiety, facilitating more intuitive eating.

The Mind-Body Connection in Eating Habits

The intricate connection between the mind and body plays a pivotal role in our eating habits. The mind-body connection refers to the interplay between psychological factors, such as thoughts and emotions, and physiological responses within the body. This connection profoundly influences our relationship with food, determining not only what we eat but also how our bodies respond to the nutrients we consume.

Consider the experience of stress eating – a common phenomenon where emotions trigger overconsumption of certain foods, often high in sugar and fat. This reaction stems from the mind-body connection; stress triggers the release of cortisol, a hormone that can lead to increased appetite and cravings for comfort foods. Mindful eating addresses this connection by encouraging individuals to recognize their emotional triggers and respond with awareness, breaking the automatic response cycle.

Psychological Benefits of Mindful Eating

Mindful eating engenders a cascade of psychological benefits that extend far beyond the immediate act of eating. By fostering an awareness of thoughts, emotions, and bodily sensations during meals, individuals develop a greater understanding of their relationship with food and their inner selves.

Practicing mindfulness while eating cultivates a heightened sense of presence, allowing individuals to savor the sensory experience of each bite. This increased sensory awareness counteracts mindless overeating, a common consequence of eating while distracted. As individuals learn to fully engage with their meals, they naturally become more attuned to their body's cues of fullness, ultimately promoting healthier portion control.

Additionally, mindful eating encourages a shift in mindset from self-judgment to self-compassion. By adopting a non-judgmental attitude towards their eating habits, individuals can dismantle the cycle of guilt and shame that often accompanies dietary choices. This practice of self-compassion extends beyond the dinner table, contributing to improved self-esteem and reduced stress levels.

Physiological Benefits of Mindful Eating

The physiological benefits of mindful eating are equally compelling. One of the most significant impacts lies in improved digestion. When we eat in a rushed or stressed state, the body activates the sympathetic nervous system – the "fight or flight" response. This state hinders optimal digestion, leading to discomfort, bloating, and other digestive issues.

Conversely, practicing mindfulness activates the parasympathetic nervous system – the "rest and digest" mode. This shift facilitates better digestion and nutrient absorption, minimizing gastrointestinal discomfort. Furthermore, mindful eating promotes slower chewing and thorough mastication, aiding the digestive process and preventing issues like indigestion.

Conclusion

The science behind mindful eating underscores its legitimacy as a holistic approach to well-being. With a foundation rooted in empirical research, mindful eating harnesses the profound mind-body connection that shapes our eating habits. By integrating mindfulness into our dietary practices, we unlock psychological benefits that reshape our relationship with food – from heightened sensory experiences to increased self-compassion. Simultaneously, the physiological advantages of mindful eating promote improved digestion and overall physical comfort.

As science continues to unveil the transformative potential of mindful eating, its relevance extends far beyond individual health. It touches on broader societal issues like obesity, disordered eating, and the cultural norms surrounding food consumption. Ultimately, the science of mindful eating invites us to reevaluate our approach to nourishment, promoting a harmonious dance between mindfulness and nourishment that nurtures our bodies, minds, and spirits.

CHAPTER THREE

Getting Started: Setting Intentions and Goals for a Transformative 30-Day Mindful Eating Challenge

Embarking on a 30-day mindful eating challenge marks the initiation of a profound journey towards a more conscious and balanced relationship with food. As we delve into this endeavor, the foundation we lay through setting intentions and goals becomes pivotal to our success. This phase is not just about dietary shifts; it's about embracing a holistic transformation that encompasses our mind, body, and spirit. Guiding readers through the process of setting intentions, defining meaningful goals, and cultivating lasting motivation, this exploration equips individuals with the tools they need to embark on a journey of mindful eating with purpose and perseverance.

Setting Intentions: The Heart of Mindful Eating

Intentions serve as the guiding lights that illuminate our path. They encapsulate the essence of our desires, aspirations, and reasons for engaging in the mindful eating challenge. Setting intentions for the journey involves tapping into our innermost motivations, reflecting on our current relationship with food, and envisioning the transformative potential of the next 30 days.

Begin by carving out a quiet space for introspection. Consider your reasons for embarking on this journey – is it to foster a healthier relationship with food, to reconnect with your body's signals, or to cultivate a sense of mindful awareness in all aspects of life? Your intentions are deeply personal and can span physical, emotional, and spiritual dimensions.

Write down your intentions in a journal or on a piece of paper. Keep them concise and specific, allowing them to resonate deeply within you. By anchoring your journey with clear intentions, you create a powerful sense of purpose that will guide you through the challenges and triumphs that lie ahead.

Defining Realistic and Meaningful Goals

Intentions provide the overarching direction, while goals break down the journey into actionable steps. When defining goals for your mindful eating challenge, it's essential to strike a balance between ambition and feasibility. Setting overly ambitious goals can lead to frustration, while setting goals that are too easy might not stimulate growth.

Start by assessing your current habits and identifying areas you wish to transform. Are you prone to emotional eating? Do you struggle with portion control? Are you seeking to enhance your awareness of hunger and satiety cues? Tailor your goals to address these specific aspects of your relationship with food.

Make your goals SMART – Specific, Measurable, Achievable, Relevant, and Time-bound. For instance, if emotional eating is a challenge, a SMART goal could be: "I will practice mindful breathing for 5 minutes before each meal to create space between emotions and eating for the next 30 days."

Strategies for Sustaining Motivation

The path of any transformative journey is marked by both peaks and valleys. Staying motivated throughout the 30-day mindful eating challenge requires cultivating a resilient mindset and implementing strategies to navigate obstacles.

1. Create a Supportive Environment: Surround yourself with like-minded individuals who share your journey. Join online communities, find an accountability partner, or inform friends and family about your challenge. Having a support system

bolsters your motivation and provides a space to share experiences.

2. Practice Self-Compassion: Progress is rarely linear. There might be days when old habits resurface or challenges seem insurmountable. Instead of self-criticism, approach setbacks with self-compassion. Treat yourself with the same kindness you would offer a friend facing a similar situation.

3. Track Progress: Keep a journal to document your journey. Note moments of triumph, insights gained, and challenges overcome. Tracking your progress reinforces your commitment and offers a tangible reminder of how far you've come.

4. Celebrate Small Wins: Acknowledge and celebrate the small victories along the way. Every mindful meal, each instance of choosing nourishing foods, and all moments of heightened awareness deserve recognition.

5. Practice Mindfulness Beyond Meals: Extend the principles of mindfulness to other aspects of your life. Engage in mindful breathing, meditation, or body scans to maintain a state of presence beyond

mealtimes. This continuity fosters a deeper connection to your intentions.

6. Adjust Goals as Needed: Be flexible with your goals. If you find that a particular goal isn't resonating or feels too challenging, consider adjusting it. The journey is about growth and learning, and adaptations are a natural part of that process.

7. Visualize Your Desired Outcome: Take a few moments each day to visualize the outcome you're working towards. Envision yourself embodying mindful eating habits and experiencing the positive changes you seek.

Conclusion

Setting intentions and defining goals lay the groundwork for a successful and transformative 30-day mindful eating challenge. Through these processes, you align your inner aspirations with actionable steps, creating a roadmap that leads to a more mindful and balanced relationship with food. The journey is not without its hurdles, but armed with clear intentions, meaningful goals, and strategies for maintaining motivation, you possess the tools needed to navigate the challenges and embrace the triumphs that await. As you embark on this path of self-discovery and mindful awareness, remember that every step forward is a testament to your dedication to well-being and the transformation that lies within your grasp.

CHAPTER FOUR

Mindful Eating Practices: Savoring the Experience of Nourishment

In a world that often encourages rushed and distracted eating, the practice of mindful eating emerges as a gentle reminder to savor the simple yet profound act of nourishing our bodies. Beyond being a dietary regimen, mindful eating is a transformative approach that invites us to engage all our senses, immerse ourselves in the present moment, and cultivate a deeper connection with the food we consume. This exploration delves into the art of mindful eating practices, unveiling specific techniques, emphasizing sensory engagement, and providing exercises that allow readers to embark on a journey of heightened awareness and appreciation for the flavors, textures, and aromas that grace their plates.

Specific Techniques for Practicing Mindful Eating

Mindful eating transcends the realm of passive consumption. It invites us to be active participants in the nourishment process, engaging our attention and awareness in every bite. The following techniques lay the foundation for mindful eating practices:

1. Slow Down: Begin by slowing down the pace of your eating. Put your utensils down between bites, take a breath, and savor the flavors before taking another bite. This deliberate pacing allows you to fully experience each mouthful.

2. Engage Your Senses: Consciously engage all your senses – sight, smell, touch, taste, and even sound – while eating. Observe the colors and textures of your food, inhale the aromas, feel the textures on your tongue, and listen to the sounds of each bite.

3. Turn Off Distractions: Minimize distractions by turning off screens, putting away phones, and creating a dedicated space for eating. This practice ensures that your focus remains on the experience of eating.

4. Practice Gratitude: Before you begin your meal, take a moment to express gratitude for the food on your plate. Acknowledge the effort that went into its production and the journey it took to reach your table.

5. Chew Thoroughly: Chew each bite thoroughly, savoring the flavors as they unfold. This not only

enhances digestion but also allows you to fully experience the taste and texture of the food.

6. Check In with Hunger and Satiety: Pause midway through your meal to check in with your body's hunger and satiety cues. Ask yourself how hungry you are and how satisfied you feel. This practice prevents overeating and fosters a mindful connection to your body's needs.

Engaging All the Senses During Meals

Sensory engagement lies at the heart of mindful eating, transforming a mundane act into a multisensory experience that brings depth and richness to each bite. By involving all our senses, we enhance our connection to the present moment and elevate our appreciation for the food before us.

- Sight: Take a moment to visually appreciate the presentation of your meal. Notice the colors, arrangement, and visual appeal of the food on your plate. This initial observation sets the stage for a mindful dining experience.

- Smell: Inhale the aromas that waft from your plate. Close your eyes for a moment and allow the scents to evoke memories, feelings, and associations. This sensory engagement enhances the anticipation of flavors to come.

- Touch: Use your fingers or utensils to explore the textures of your food. Notice the variations in temperature, consistency, and surface. Pay attention to the tactile sensations as you lift, cut, and grasp each morsel.

- Taste: As you bring the food to your mouth, allow it to linger on your tongue. Gently move it around, exploring the different taste receptors that detect sweet, salty, sour, bitter, and umami flavors.

- Sound: Listen to the sounds your food makes as you bite into it. Whether it's the crisp crunch of a vegetable or the delicate sound of a fork against a plate, these auditory cues add another layer of sensory experience.

Exercises to Cultivate Deeper Appreciation

Cultivating a deeper appreciation for the flavors and textures of your food requires intention and practice. Here are exercises that encourage a heightened sensory connection during meals:

1. The Five-Minute Bite: Choose a single bite of food and spend five minutes engaging all your senses

with it. Observe its appearance, inhale its aroma, touch its textures, taste its flavors, and savor its journey from plate to palate.

2. Blindfolded Tasting: Blindfold yourself and have someone place small, varied bites of food on your plate. Engage your senses without the visual cues, allowing your taste buds, nose, and touch to guide your experience.

3. Mindful Gratitude: Before eating, take a moment to express gratitude for the journey the food has taken – from seed to plate. Reflect on the efforts of farmers, producers, and all those involved in bringing the meal to your table.

4. Texture Exploration: Choose a meal with a variety of textures. Pay close attention to how each texture feels in your mouth – the crunch, the smoothness, the chewiness. Allow yourself to fully embrace the tactile sensations.

5. Sensory Journaling: Maintain a sensory journal to document your mindful eating experiences. Describe the sensory aspects of each meal, including the colors, aromas, textures, and tastes. This practice heightens your awareness over time.

Conclusion

Mindful eating practices beckon us to return to the essence of nourishment – to immerse ourselves fully in the sensory symphony that unfolds with every meal. Engaging all our senses during meals transforms eating from a routine chore into a moment of mindful presence, fostering a deeper connection with our food and our bodies. Through specific techniques, sensory engagement, and purposeful exercises, we elevate the act of eating to an art form that nurtures not only our physical bodies but also our emotional and spiritual selves. As we embark on this journey of savoring the experience, we embrace a richer, more conscious relationship with food that invites us to be fully present, one bite at a time.

CHAPTER FIVE

Unraveling Emotional Eating: Navigating the Connection Between Emotions and Food

Food, beyond its role as sustenance, often becomes a canvas onto which we paint our emotions, seeking solace, comfort, or distraction. This intricate dance between emotions and eating habits is what defines emotional eating – a phenomenon deeply ingrained in our relationship with food. While occasionally turning to food for emotional relief is natural, unchecked emotional eating can lead to a cycle of unhealthy habits and imbalanced well-being. To unveil the layers of emotional eating, empower readers to identify triggers, and provide effective coping strategies, this exploration delves into the intersection of emotions and food, offering insights and mindfulness exercises that pave the way for a healthier and more mindful approach to eating.

The Role of Emotions in Our Eating Habits

Food and emotions share a complex interplay that has its roots in our human experience. From celebrations laden with feasts to comforting childhood memories centered around favorite treats, food becomes intertwined with our emotions from an early age. Emotional eating occurs when we turn to food not out of physical hunger but as a response to emotional triggers – stress, sadness, anxiety, boredom, or even happiness.

Emotions can influence our food choices in several ways:

- Comfort: Seeking comfort in familiar foods when feeling down or stressed.
- Reward: Using indulgent foods as rewards for achievements or as a way to celebrate.
- Distraction: Turning to food as a way to avoid or distract from uncomfortable emotions.
- Cravings: Experiencing strong cravings for specific foods in response to emotional states.

Identifying Triggers for Emotional Eating and Developing Coping Strategies

Recognizing emotional eating patterns begins with self-awareness. Identifying triggers helps illuminate the emotional landscape that influences our food choices. Triggers can vary from person to person and may encompass:

- Stress: Pressures from work, relationships, or other life challenges.
- Emotional States: Sadness, loneliness, anxiety, or frustration.

- Boredom: Lack of stimulation or purpose leading to mindless eating.
- Social Situations: Social gatherings or peer pressure influencing food choices.
- Habitual Responses: Associating certain emotions with specific foods due to past experiences.

Once triggers are identified, building a toolbox of coping strategies becomes crucial. Here are effective strategies to navigate emotional triggers:

1. Mindful Pause: Before reaching for food, take a moment to pause. Engage in deep breathing or a brief mindfulness exercise to create space between the emotion and the impulse to eat.

2. Emotion Journaling: Keep an emotion journal to log your emotional states throughout the day. This practice heightens awareness of patterns and correlations between emotions and eating.

3. Distract and Delay: Engage in activities that distract from the immediate urge to eat. Read a book, take a walk, or practice a hobby before revisiting the decision to eat.

4. Create a Support System: Reach out to friends, family, or support groups when you're struggling

with emotional triggers. Connecting with others can provide comfort and alleviate the need for emotional eating.

5. Mindful Eating Practices: Incorporate mindfulness techniques into your meals. Engage all your senses, eat slowly, and savor the experience. This practice cultivates awareness and prevents mindless eating.

Mindfulness Exercises to Enhance Emotional Awareness and Regulation

Mindfulness serves as a potent tool to unravel emotional eating patterns. By cultivating an awareness of our emotions without judgment, we can create a space for conscious responses rather than reactive ones. The following exercises enhance emotional awareness and regulation:

1. Body Scan Meditation: Dedicate a few minutes each day to a body scan meditation. Start at your toes and slowly move your attention upward, noticing any physical sensations or tension. This practice connects you to your body and its emotional signals.

2. Emotion Labeling: Throughout the day, pause to label your emotions. Use descriptive words like

"anxious," "happy," or "frustrated." This practice creates a mental distance from the emotion, allowing you to observe without immediate reaction.

3. Breath Awareness: When facing emotional triggers, turn to your breath. Inhale and exhale mindfully, counting each breath. This technique grounds you in the present moment and calms the nervous system.

4. R.A.I.N. Technique: R.A.I.N. stands for Recognize, Allow, Investigate, and Non-identify. When an emotion arises, recognize it, allow it to be present, investigate its sensations, and release any identification with it.

Conclusion

Unraveling emotional eating is a journey of self-discovery that invites us to explore the intricate dance between our emotions and our relationship with food. By identifying triggers, developing coping strategies, and integrating mindfulness exercises, we transform emotional eating from a reactive habit into a conscious and empowered choice. This process not only nurtures a healthier relationship with food but also fosters emotional well-being and resilience. As we navigate this exploration, we gain the tools to navigate our emotions with grace and compassion, choosing nourishment that nurtures both body and soul.

CHAPTER SIX

Overcoming Challenges and Roadblocks: Navigating the Mindful Eating Journey with Resilience

The path of mindful eating, though transformative and empowering, is not without its challenges. As individuals embark on this journey to cultivate a healthier and more conscious relationship with food, they encounter various obstacles that can test their resolve and commitment. From cravings that seem insurmountable to the pressures of social situations that challenge mindful choices, these hurdles can deter progress. However, armed with strategies, insights, and a foundation of resilience, individuals can not only overcome these challenges but also emerge stronger, more self-aware, and better equipped to navigate the complexities of the mindful eating journey.

Common Obstacles in the Mindful Eating Journey

1. Cravings: Cravings often stem from habit, emotional triggers, or conditioned responses to specific cues. These powerful urges can challenge mindful eating intentions.

2. Social Pressures: Social gatherings, peer influence, and cultural norms can lead to eating choices that conflict with mindful intentions.

3. Mindless Eating Habits: Breaking the cycle of mindless eating – driven by distractions, haste, or boredom – requires consistent effort.

4. Setbacks and Slip-Ups: It's natural to experience setbacks or slip-ups on the journey. These instances can trigger feelings of guilt or self-doubt.

5. Emotional Eating: Emotional states such as stress, sadness, or anxiety can lead to impulsive and emotionally driven eating habits.

Strategies for Dealing with Challenges

1. Cravings:

- Pause and Reflect: When a craving arises, pause and reflect on its origin. Is it driven by hunger or emotion? Acknowledging the craving's source can empower mindful choices.

- Delayed Gratification: Tell yourself you'll revisit the craving in 15 minutes. This delay can often mitigate its intensity, allowing you to make a more conscious decision.

2. Social Pressures:

   - Communicate: Inform friends and family about your mindful eating journey. Their understanding can reduce pressure and provide a supportive environment.

   - Plan Ahead: Before social events, mentally prepare by visualizing making mindful choices. Identify healthy options available and set your intention.

3. Mindless Eating Habits:

   - Create Rituals: Establish mindful eating rituals, such as setting the table, taking a few deep breaths before eating, or practicing gratitude.

4. Setbacks and Slip-Ups:

   - Practice Self-Compassion: Approach setbacks with self-compassion rather than self-criticism. Remember that progress is nonlinear, and every step counts.

5. Emotional Eating:

   - Mindful Pause: When emotions trigger eating urges, pause and take a few deep breaths. Observe the emotions without judgment before deciding to eat.

Building Resilience and Maintaining Progress

1.   Self-Reflection: Regularly   engage   in self-reflection to assess your progress, challenges, and areas for growth. Journaling can be a valuable tool for this practice.

2. Support System: Surround yourself with individuals who understand and support your mindful eating journey. Connect with friends, family, or online communities for encouragement.

3. Mindful Awareness: Continuously cultivate mindful awareness not only during meals but throughout daily life. Engage in practices like mindful breathing or body scans to stay present.

4. Goal Adaptation: Be flexible with your goals. If a certain goal becomes too challenging or no longer resonates, adapt it to align with your evolving needs.

5. Celebrate Progress: Celebrate even the smallest victories along the way. Acknowledge the moments when you choose mindfulness over habit, fostering a positive outlook.

6. Mindful Eating Rituals: Develop consistent mindful eating rituals that serve as anchors in your

journey. These rituals reinforce your commitment and provide stability.

Guidance on Building Resilience

1. Developing Mindful Habits:
   - Start Small: Focus on incorporating one mindful habit at a time. Gradual changes are more sustainable and effective.

2. Mindful Breathing:
   - Deep Breathing: Engage in deep, intentional breathing exercises whenever you feel overwhelmed. This practice calms the nervous system and enhances self-awareness.

3. Mindful Awareness Practices:
   - Body Scan Meditation: Regularly practice body scan meditations to connect with physical sensations and emotional states. This fosters resilience in the face of challenges.

4. Mindful Eating Reminders:
   - Visual Cues: Place reminders in your environment – on the fridge or dining table – to prompt mindful eating awareness.

Conclusion

The mindful eating journey is a transformative path marked by both triumphs and trials. Overcoming challenges and roadblocks requires resilience, self-awareness, and a commitment to personal growth. By recognizing the common obstacles, adopting effective strategies, and building resilience, individuals can navigate the complexities of cravings, social pressures, setbacks, and emotional triggers with grace and mindfulness. Each challenge met with awareness and intention becomes an opportunity for growth, deepening the connection with oneself and fostering a more profound relationship with food. The journey's essence lies not just in the destination but in the evolution of the self along the way – a journey illuminated by mindful choices and the strength of resilience.

CHAPTER SEVEN

Beyond the 30 Days: Embracing a Lifelong Journey of Mindful Eating

Completing a 30-day mindful eating challenge marks an accomplishment, but the true transformation lies in the journey beyond those initial days. Mindful eating isn't a temporary fix or a quick diet – it's a way of life that invites individuals to engage with food and nourishment in a profound and sustainable manner. As the challenge concludes, the transition to sustaining mindful eating involves integrating mindfulness into everyday eating routines, nurturing a resilient mindset, and accessing ongoing support. This exploration delves into the art of transitioning from the challenge to a lifelong mindful eating lifestyle, offering insights, practical tips, and resources to empower individuals on their continued journey of mindful nourishment.

Transitioning to a Mindful Eating Lifestyle

The conclusion of the 30-day challenge signifies not the end but the beginning of a lifelong journey toward mindful eating. This transition involves weaving the practices, insights, and mindfulness cultivated during the challenge into the fabric of daily life. Mindful eating isn't a destination; it's a path that offers the gifts of heightened awareness, nourishment, and self-compassion.

Tips for Integrating Mindfulness into Everyday Eating Routines

1. Start Small: Begin by choosing one meal or snack each day to practice mindful eating. Gradually expand the practice to other meals as you feel comfortable.

2. Set Intentions: Prior to each meal, take a moment to set an intention for mindful eating. This simple ritual helps you approach the meal with awareness.

3. Mindful Moments: Infuse moments of mindfulness throughout the day. Pause for a few deep breaths before eating, and take a moment to express gratitude for your food.

4. Mindful Grocery Shopping: Approach grocery shopping with mindfulness. Make a shopping list, choose whole and nourishing foods, and consider the origins of what you're purchasing.

5. Create a Mindful Eating Space: Designate a specific space for eating, free from distractions.

This space can serve as a reminder to engage fully with your meals.

6. Practice Portion Control: Pay attention to portion sizes and honor your body's signals of hunger and fullness. Eating mindfully includes being attuned to your body's needs.

7. Chew Thoroughly: Chew each bite slowly and thoroughly. This not only enhances digestion but also allows you to savor the flavors and textures of your food.

8. Engage Your Senses: Continuously engage all your senses during meals. Savor the aromas, textures, and tastes, allowing yourself to fully experience each bite.

Nurturing a Resilient Mindset

Maintaining a lifelong mindful eating practice requires nurturing a mindset of resilience, self-compassion, and patience. As you encounter challenges and moments of imperfection, remember that mindful eating is a journey, not a destination. Here are ways to foster a resilient mindset:

1. Embrace Imperfection: Acknowledge that mindful eating is a practice, and there will be moments when you slip into old habits. Approach these moments with self-compassion rather than self-criticism.

2. Cultivate Self-Awareness: Continuously cultivate self-awareness to identify patterns, triggers, and reactions that impact your eating habits. This awareness allows you to make conscious choices.

3. Celebrate Progress: Acknowledge and celebrate your progress – no matter how small. Celebrate every moment of mindfulness and self-awareness as a step toward a more balanced relationship with food.

4. Mindful Reflection: Regularly reflect on the impact of mindful eating on your well-being. Notice the physical, emotional, and psychological changes that arise from this practice.

Ongoing Support and Further Exploration

As you transition to a lifelong mindful eating lifestyle, it's important to have access to ongoing support and resources that can enrich your journey:

1.   Mindfulness   Meditation   Apps: Utilize mindfulness meditation apps that offer guided meditations and mindfulness exercises to deepen your practice.

2. Mindful Eating Books: Explore books on mindful eating that provide in-depth insights, practical exercises, and real-life stories to inspire and guide your journey.

3. Online Communities: Join online forums or social media groups focused on mindful eating. These communities provide a space to connect with like-minded individuals, share experiences, and seek advice.

4. Mindful Eating Workshops and Retreats: Attend workshops, seminars, or retreats that delve deeper into mindful eating practices. These immersive experiences offer an opportunity for learning and growth.

5.   Mindfulness   Teachers: Consider   seeking guidance   from   mindfulness   teachers   or practitioners who can offer personalized support and guidance tailored to your journey.

6. Journaling: Continue journaling about your mindful eating experiences. Documenting your thoughts, challenges, and triumphs can provide valuable insights over time.

Conclusion

The journey of mindful eating extends far beyond the initial 30 days, guiding individuals toward a lifelong path of self-awareness, nourishment, and well-being. By integrating mindfulness into everyday eating routines, nurturing a resilient mindset, and accessing ongoing support, individuals embark on a transformative journey that celebrates food as a source of nourishment for both body and soul. Mindful eating becomes not just a practice but a way of life – a journey that unfolds with each conscious bite, fostering a deeper connection to oneself, the food we consume, and the world around us. As you embrace this lifelong journey, remember that every moment of mindfulness is a step toward lasting change and a more mindful, balanced, and fulfilling relationship with food.